40
Prayers for Dementia Caregivers

By
Diane McGiffin LPN
Marlene Graeve RN
D. Duane Engler

Psalm 46:1

God is our refuge and strength, an ever present help in trouble. NIV

God is our refuge and strength, a tested help in times of trouble. TLB

Galatians 6:9

Let us not become weary in doing good, for at the proper time we will reap a harvest if we do not give up. NIV

And let us not get tired of doing what is right, for after a while we will reap a harvest of blessing if we don't get discouraged and give up. TLB

40 Prayers for Dementia Caregivers is Copyright © 2014 D. Duane Engler

Diane McGiffen, Marlene Graeve are expert contributors to this series.

40 Prayers™ Series and 40 Christian Prayers™ Series are registered by D. Duane Engler © 2014

Quote on book cover is from Amazon reviewer regarding 40 Prayers for Christmas review in 2013.

All rights reserved.

No portion of this book may be reproduced, stored in a retrieval system, or transmitted in any form or by any means (electronic, mechanical, photocopy, recording, or any other medium) without the express written permission of the author. Please email the author at engler21@gmail.com

Bible translations have variances, limitations, and nuances. The New International Version (NIV) and The Living Bible (TLB) versions are used in this book. Two versions are included to provide a different perspective, deepen your understanding of the verse, and strengthen your journey with Christ Other Bible versions are available at www.biblegateway.org.

Unless noted all Bible verses are from the following sources.

The Holy Bible, New International Version®, NIV® Copyright 1973, 1978, 1984, 2011 by Biblica, Inc. ™ Used by permission. All rights reserved worldwide.

Scripture taken from *The Message*. Copyright © 1993, 1994, 1995, 1996, 2000, 2001, 2002. Used by permission of NavPress Publishing Group.

Scripture quotations marked (TLB) are from The Living Bible copyright © 1971. Used by permission of Tyndale House Publishers, Inc., Wheaton, IL 60189. All rights reserved.

Other titles by D. Duane Engler at Amazon.com

The Christian Revival Diet™ © 2013

Numerous Titles in the 40 Prayers™ Series © 2013 and the 40 Christian Prayers™ Series

40 by 40: 40 Short Stories with Less Than 40 Words © 2013

40 Prayers and Proverbs™

40 Prayers and Psalms™

Other books by Dr. Bett Mickels & D. Duane Engler

40 Prayers for Entrepreneurs

40 Prayers When God Says Wait

40 Prayers During Suffering and Tragedy

Additional books coming soon.

Table of Contents

Table of Contents
Introduction
#1 Uncertainty
#2 Lean Not
#3 The Lord's Hand
#4 Facts Versus The Unseen
#5 Abound in Hope
#6 The Lord's Child
#7 Clinging to Your Promises
#8 Victory
#9 On Overload
#10 Alongside
#11 You Do Not Know
#12 Mercy
#13 The Long View
#14 Shine
#15 Thy Will
#16 Opportunity
#17 Promises
#18 Unexpected Blessings
#19 Obedience
#20 Prayer for Refuge
#21 My Fortress
#22 Broaden the Path
#23 To Feel Whole
#24 Wasteful Worry
#25 Knit Me Together
#26 The Word Holy
#27 My Quiet Time
#28 Less of me, More of You

#29 Yoked to You

#30 A Contagious Smile

#31 Obedience to God

#32 Call to Me

#33 When I am Weak, I am Strong

#34 Wait!

#35 God is For Us!

#36 Where Does My Help Come From

#37 God Provides

#38 The Lord, the Great Physician

#39 A Cheerful Heart

#40 Guide Me, O Lord

About The Authors

Scripture Meditation and Prayer

Author's Section on Prayer and the 40 Prayers™ Series:

Introduction

There is a universal need for care with aging, illness and dying. Yet, there is a special approach, an expertise, a certain understanding needed when caring for a loved one with dementia. The definition of dementia by the Alzheimer's Association is a general term for a decline in mental ability severe enough to interfere with daily life. It is not one specific disease but is a result of a number of causative factors--the main one being Alzheimer's disease. This book of prayers is written specifically for those individuals who find themselves caring for a loved one suffering from dementia.

Compassionate care-giving takes many forms. You might be a 24/7 in-home primary support person or one who is on call by phone for assistance. You might provide transportation to doctor appointments or to the grocery store. Perhaps you attend care conference meetings once a quarter and are required to make decisions that will affect your loved one. You are a caregiver! Some family members do not realize they are caregivers. They simply consider themselves family members caring for their loved one as would be expected of any family member or friend. Call it what you will, but care-giving is a special calling--one that needs positive encouragement-- and where does one go for that?

Thank God, there are friends and family that walk alongside. Respite may be an option for a long-awaited vacation. There are tools and medications that might alleviate symptoms and undesirable behaviors.

However, amidst the exhaustion, the frustrations, the overwhelming uncertainties of it all, who is there to help? Who can alleviate your weariness and help you bear this heavy burden? There may have been no discernible improvements in any avenue of daily care for months on end. Who is it who understands how you feel? Our creator is the only one who fully understands. He is our refuge, our strength, our help in time of trouble. His name is Jesus. Is it ever possible to obtain a modicum of peace while living the chaotic, disorganized role of care-giver to a loved one with an impaired memory? Only Jesus can transform our lives and strengthen us to be victorious over our circumstances. Happiness is a transient thing, but true joy comes from within like a light that fills you. This joy comes from knowing Jesus and his promise to uphold us. He has said He is the Light of the world. Better to live with a light to shine on our path than to stumble in the darkness.

There is only one way to really get to know Jesus and that is through His Holy Word. The Bible and the verses we cling to can strengthen us in ways we never imagined. We are created to thrive and live victoriously--not just cope to get through the day. The Word of God is powerful. Plant these verses you will find in these 40 prayers deep in your heart and hang onto the wisdom of the words of God. In repeating the words, we are speaking as God speaks. Therein lies the wisdom, the holiness, the sharing in God's glory. The Holy of all Holies is always with you, helping you in this most difficult situation to find a peace this world may never know.

"Peace I leave with you, my peace I give to you. I do not give to you as the world gives. Do not let your hearts be troubled, and do not let them be afraid." John 13:27

Respectfully offered,
Diane McGiffin LPN, Marlene Graeve RN, D. Duane Engler

40 Prayers For Dementia Caregivers

#1 Uncertainty

There is a glimmer of improvement, then there is a crashing downward spiral of offensive behavior. There is a clear concise articulated sentence, then there is a sentence of mumble jumble. There is a hearty laugh reminding me of the good old days, then there is a period of crying and depressed statements. This is how the days develop as I care for my loved one with dementia. This ambivalence finds me in a constant state of uncertainty. I never know what tomorrow will bring. Stress is upon me. Peace is what I long for. I know nothing compares to the promises I have in You, Jesus. You promise to be with me. In fact you say you will go before me, walk along beside me and cover my back. This gives me peace. My life is in the hands of the king that is unlike any other king. The king of all kings. This gives me a peace that does not come from my day to day world.

Revelations 17:14

They will wage war against the Lamb, but the Lamb will triumph over them because he is Lord of lords and King of kings—and with him will be his called, chosen and faithful followers. NIV

Together they will wage war against the Lamb, and the Lamb will conquer them; for he is Lord over all lords, and King of kings, and his people are the called and chosen and faithful ones. TLB

40 Prayers For Dementia Caregivers

#2 Lean Not

Heavenly Father, how is it that some people just thrive and flourish even into old age? They have boundless energy and resources. They have their families. They have their health. They have their minds, their dignity, their sense of self. I try and try but I can't understand how or why this has happened. We were quite the pair, he and I, weren't we Lord? Our life was good and we were thankful.

Foolishly, we thought it would go on and on. Then came that day. That diagnosis. That word. We managed for a while until he began to slip away from me. We sought answers, Lord, but You and Your Word are the only answer we can count on. We found that out. Father, we must continue to draw close to You and have You lead us according to Your will. Only You can take us to where we need to be.

Proverbs 3: 5-6

Trust in the LORD with all your heart and lean not on your own understanding; in all your ways submit to him, and he will make your paths straight. NIV

If you want favor with both God and man, and a reputation for good judgment and common sense, then trust the Lord completely; don't ever trust yourself. In everything you do, put God first, and he will direct you and crown your efforts with success. TLB

40 Prayers For Dementia Caregivers

#3 The Lord's Hand

Heavenly Father, sometimes this burden is too much to bear. This man who was a giant to me, who could handle anything that came his way, now has trouble remembering who I am. Oh yes, he knows he loves me; he just can't remember my name. How can this be? Some days I think my heart is actually breaking. I beg you to give me strength. Help me to make informed and wise decisions for him.

Where once he made decisions for me, I now must make them for him. Lord, please give me the perseverance and fortitude to guide him along this path, this difficult road home. Until he reaches the safety of Your arms, uphold us both.

Oh Father, use my life to Your glory and honor.

Isaiah 41:10

So do not fear, for I am with you; do not be dismayed, for I am your God. I will strengthen you and help you; I will uphold you with my righteous right hand. NIV

Fear not, for I am with you. Do not be dismayed. I am your God. I will strengthen you; I will help you; I will uphold you with my victorious right hand. TLB

40 Prayers For Dementia Caregivers

#4 Facts Versus The Unseen

How does this organ function? Lord, who can fathom the intricacies of the brain? How many times have I sat down with books, diagrams, professional journals? How many doctors and scientist have I consulted? How many care conferences have I attended? Father, day in and out, my profession is to solve problems. Critical thinking. That is what I thought I did well. Why can't I help him? He was there for me my entire life. Now he needs me and I am unable to do anything. I feel helpless and ineffective.

Only you, Lord, see and understand. He professed his faith as far back as I can remember. I, with my advanced degrees, looked on from an intellectual distance. Now, Father, I fully comprehend what he was trying, in his gracious way, to explain-that with all my education, I did not know it all. There are more things unseen than those that are seen. I have been attempting to save him, while all the time he was preparing the way, to save me.

2 Corinthians 4:16-18

Therefore we do not lose heart. Though outwardly we are wasting away, yet inwardly we are being renewed day by day. For our light and momentary troubles are achieving for us an eternal glory that far outweighs them all. So we fix our eyes not on what is seen, but on what is unseen, since what is seen is temporary, but what is unseen is eternal. .NIV

That is why we never give up. Though our bodies are dying, our inner strength in the Lord is growing every day. These troubles and sufferings of ours are, after all, quite small and won't last very long. Yet this short time of distress will result in God's richest blessing upon us forever and ever! So we do not look at what we can see right now, the troubles all around us, but we look forward to the joys in heaven which we have not yet seen. The troubles will soon be over, but the joys to come will last forever. TLB

#5 Abound in Hope

Oh Father, who could ever have predicted this? We thought we were doing all the right things to protect ourselves against all types of diseases. Now there are so many things he is unable to do. Admittedly, some may seem small, but they are important to him. His sense of dignity is being whittled away.

Father help me to help him without having him feel less than he is. Give me strength and motivation to be a gracious caregiver that is sensitive to his feelings of worth. Good humor and patience is what I need to get through this difficult day. We need your healing spirit Lord to be able to hang onto our hope. Without hope, discouragement sets in, and my joy is gone.

Romans 15:13

May the God of hope fill you with all joy and peace as you trust in him, so that you may overflow with hope by the power of the Holy Spirit. NIV

So I pray for you Gentiles that God who gives you hope will keep you happy and full of peace as you believe in him. I pray that God will help you overflow with hope in him through the Holy Spirit's power within you. TLB

40 Prayers For Dementia Caregivers

#6 The Lord's Child

Father, as I drive along on this perfect day you have created, I can't help but feel happy and blessed. I am in the prime of my life and I feel well. Yet Lord, I know this is not true for the one you have entrusted to my care. He is broken and vulnerable. Heavenly Father, help me to do my best.

Guide my hands, my heart, and my mind. Give me eyes to see the person, not the physical and cognitive deficits. Let me see the person who yet has value -- A child of God who continues to be well loved.

Proverbs 16:3

Commit to the LORD whatever you do, and he will establish your plans. NIV

Commit your work to the Lord, then it will succeed. TLB

40 Prayers For Dementia Caregivers

#7 Clinging to Your Promises

Lord, I have no one with whom I can share this burden. I need You. I place my trust in You. I realize everyone has trials. How can I accept your wondrous gifts then turn away from You when the storms of life threaten? It is exactly now, at this time, I need to feel your Holy Spirit surrounding me.

Envelop me in Your love. Father I don't understand the reason for this. Is there something I am to learn from this sorrow? I feel uncertain. But I do have your promises! I cling to Your word.

Romans 8:28

And we know that in all things God works for the good of those who love him, who[a] have been called according to his purpose. NIV

And we know that all that happens to us is working for our good if we love God and are fitting into his plans. TLB

40 Prayers For Dementia Caregivers

#8 Victory

Father God, do you remember when he spoke five languages? Of course You do, just as you knew him before time began. You loved him before I met him; You made him the unique individual he was.

Father, now he is slipping away, slowly, very slowly. I am aware of the changes, and I can barely think of the anguish we may have ahead of us. Lord remain with us. Help us to navigate these troubled waters with your guidance. Lord grant me your peace.

.

John 16:33

I have told you these things, so that in me you may have peace. In this world you will have trouble. But take heart! I have overcome the world. NIV

I have told you all this so that you will have peace of heart and mind. Here on earth you will have many trials and sorrows; but cheer up, for I have overcome the world. TLB

40 Prayers For Dementia Caregivers

#9 On Overload

Lord, I can barely speak. My brain is on overload. I need to sleep but must remain vigilant. Are the doors locked? Are the car keys in a safe place? Whatever happened? How did my calm life come to this place? The changes seem fast, and yet I know well the years have passed.

Lord I call out to you. I feel unable to communicate with you coherently, but I know I can place my trust in You. I know you have a plan that is working to our good.

Jeremiah 33:3

Call to me and I will answer you and tell you great and unsearchable things you do not know. NIV

Ask me and I will tell you some remarkable secrets about what is going to happen here. TLB

40 Prayers For Dementia Caregivers

#10 Alongside

Father, you know my heart. You know my struggles day after day. You know at times I am overcome with self-pity and bitterness, longing and regret. Yet you don't abandon me. You forgive me when I ask you to forgive me for these dark thoughts. You continue to hold both me and my loved one in the palm of your hand.

Help me that I don't become so immersed in my own anguish that I fail to notice the pain of others. Father in Heaven, allow me to become a beacon to those around me, reflecting your light and love.

2 Corinthians 1:4

All praise to the God and Father of our Master, Jesus the Messiah! Father of all mercy! God of all healing counsel! He comes alongside us when we go through hard times, and before you know it, he brings us alongside someone else who is going through hard times so that we can be there for that person just as God was there for us. We have plenty of hard times that come from following the Messiah, but no more so than the good times of his healing comfort—we get a full measure of that, too. MSG

What a wonderful God we have—he is the Father of our Lord Jesus Christ, the source of every mercy, and the one who so wonderfully comforts and strengthens us in our hardships and trials. And why does he do this? So that when others are troubled, needing our sympathy and encouragement, we can pass on to them this same help and comfort God has given us. You can be sure that the more we undergo sufferings for Christ, the more he will shower us with his comfort and encouragement. TLB

40 Prayers For Dementia Caregivers

#11 You Do Not Know

Father, what miracles you have wrought. There is no one greater than you. Who else could have created this vast universe with all its complexities? As you promised in your Word, you have made your works visible for all to see. I just need to look. I need to listen. I know Lord, you have planned everything. Though these circumstances are not within my understanding, I will trust. I am passing through. One day this heartbreak will end, and all will be made clear. I will continue to pray.

Ecclesiastes 11:5
As you do not know the path of the wind, or how the body is formed in a mother's womb, so you cannot understand the work of God, the Maker of all things. NIV

God's ways are as mysterious as the pathway of the wind and as the manner in which a human spirit is infused into the little body of a baby while it is yet in its mother's womb. TLB

40 Prayers For Dementia Caregivers

#12 Mercy

Oh Father, I feel so alone. I ask for your guidance. Where once we were a team, sharing in all decisions, now it is I who must decide for both of us. How can I do it? I do not feel prepared. I still need him but he is gone from me. Decision-making skills no longer exist. Only through the wisdom and comfort of Your Word, Lord, am I able to find solace. I thank you for your unending mercy and presence.

Psalm 40:11

Do not withhold your mercy from me, LORD;
may your love and faithfulness always protect me. NIV

O Lord, don't hold back your tender mercies from me! My only hope is in your love and faithfulness. TLB

40 Prayers For Dementia Caregivers

#13 The Long View

Lord, how quickly our time passes. We're born, and in the blink of an eye we find ourselves standing on the precipice of eternity. Heavenly Father, we give praise and thanks for all the mercies You have showered upon us. We thank you for the life and love we have shared all these many years. Thank you Lord for the blessings of family and friends who have stood by us when they could have turned away. It's not an easy thing to spend a morning with someone who no longer remembers who you are. Yes, Lord, these last years have been difficult, but when viewed through the eyes of your Spirit who dwells within us and knowing the reward that lies ahead, all we can say is thank you.

1 Corinthians 15:53-55

For the perishable must clothe itself with the imperishable, and the mortal with immortality. When the perishable has been clothed with the imperishable, and the mortal with immortality, then the saying that is written will come true: "Death has been swallowed up in victory." NIV

For our earthly bodies, the ones we have now that can die, must be transformed into heavenly bodies that cannot perish but will live forever. When this happens, then at last this Scripture will come true—"Death is swallowed up in victory." O death, where then your victory? Where then your sting? TLB

40 Prayers For Dementia Caregivers

#14 Shine

Lord, I wish to manifest a cheerful countenance for all to see. Therefore, today I will not worry. I will not doubt. I will not be mortified, sad, downcast or discouraged. Instead, Lord, I will lift up my eyes. I will cast my burden upon You that I may be sustained as promised in Your Word. I will walk by faith. With your help and guidance, Lord, I can be an example of the power of Your Holy Spirit. In Jesus name, let it be so.

Matthew 5:14-16

You are the light of the world. A town built on a hill cannot be hidden. [15] Neither do people light a lamp and put it under a bowl. Instead they put it on its stand, and it gives light to everyone in the house. [16] In the same way, let your light shine before others, that they may see your good deeds and glorify your Father in heaven. NIV

You are the world's light—a city on a hill, glowing in the night for all to see. Don't hide your light! Let it shine for all; let your good deeds glow for all to see, so that they will praise your heavenly Father. TLB

#15 Thy Will

Jesus, you alone are Lord. You created the universe. You sustain it through space and time with the power of your hand. By your grace we have salvation. Lord, please, I am asking that you would grant me some understanding. Well-meaning friends tell me this shadow of his former self is Your will. I believe you have an all-encompassing plan, God, that goes far beyond what I am able to discern. He, also, had faith that you worked only for our good and not to harm us. Lord lift me up above this suffering and by your spirit allow me the courage to step out in faith to accept your will this day.

Psalm 143:10-11

Teach me to do your will, for you are my God; may your good Spirit, lead me on level ground. For your name's sake, LORD, preserve my life; in your righteousness, bring me out of trouble. NIV

Help me to do your will, for you are my God. Lead me in good paths, for your Spirit is good. Lord, saving me will bring glory to your name. Bring me out of all this trouble because you are true to your promises. TLB

40 Prayers For Dementia Caregivers

#16 Opportunity

Lord, let us seize this moment to bow our heads and sink into the comfort of your love. There are none here who can help us-none who actually comprehend what our life has become. All the doctors and nurses and social workers who have multiple initials following their names continue to profess knowledge and understanding. You and I both know, Lord, unless you have lived it, you really don't understand it.

So, Father, we choose to abide in your Love. Draw us closer during this sorrowful time. Lord, keep me from bitterness. Help me to focus on the memories of the joy we once shared. Father, I am well aware that each of us will encounter trials and burdens as we pass through this life. I am so very thankful that we have your guidance and Your Word to help see us through.

James 1:2-3

Consider it pure joy, my brothers and sisters, whenever you face trials of many kinds, because you know that the testing of your faith produces perseverance. NIV

Dear brothers, is your life full of difficulties and temptations? Then be happy, for when the way is rough, your patience has a chance to grow. TLB

40 Prayers For Dementia Caregivers

#17 Promises

Lord, sometimes I have to stop and ask myself – is this actually what has become of my life? Father, I just want to run away, to throw off all these responsibilities. I won't though, You know that Lord. Vows were made all those years ago that still hold true today. So I come to You on bended knee, Father, to beg for strength and guidance-- for an extra bit of patience and good humor just for today. I will not stray from the path. I will not give up or give in. I will, by faith, cling to your Word and the assurances You have given that one day soon all our diseases will be healed, our questions answered, and You will be waiting to welcome us into Glory, In Jesus' name.

Psalm 103:1-4

Praise the LORD, my soul;
all my inmost being, praise his holy name.
Praise the LORD, my soul,
and forget not all his benefits—
who forgives all your sins
and heals all your diseases,
who redeems your life from the pit
and crowns you with love and compassion, NIV

I bless the holy name of God with all my heart. Yes, I will bless the Lord and not forget the glorious things he does for me. He forgives all my sins. He heals me. He ransoms me from hell. He surrounds me with loving-kindness and tender mercies.
TLB

40 Prayers For Dementia Caregivers

#18 Unexpected Blessings

Lord, I now understand how blessed we are to have this opportunity to leave behind the trivial pursuits of this world and draw closer to you. Only in your Word, Father, can we find peace. We are no longer plagued with worry. We've stopped struggling and railing against our fate. Instead, each day we listen quietly for your voice. We look for wisdom in Your word. We live each day to the fullest with courage and faith, Father, knowing that you have not forgotten us – and my loved one's life is still in your gentle hands.

Psalm 27:13-14

I remain confident of this:
I will see the goodness of the LORD
in the land of the living.
Wait for the LORD;
be strong and take heart
and wait for the LORD. NIV

I am expecting the Lord to rescue me again, so that once again I will see his goodness to me here in the land of the living. Don't be impatient. Wait for the Lord, and he will come and save you! Be brave, stouthearted, and courageous. Yes, wait and he will help you. TLB

#19 Obedience

Father, even Your precious Son asked to have his cup of sorrow removed.

So, if I now beg to have this diagnosis removed from my loved one, Lord, will you think me ungrateful?

If I, with reverence, ask for a change from this, our new reality, Lord, will You think I have completely disregarded all that is good in our lives? We are frightened, Lord of these words, of these medications, of the road that looms before us. We're frightened of the unknown. Perhaps we are not looking in the right direction? Father, help us to see if there are not possibilities for new growth at this very challenging time. Help us to envision the unseen. Let us keep in our minds and hearts, always, our Lord Jesus, who after praying fervently in the garden before His hour was to come, listened quietly for Your will and was obedient even unto death.

Matthew 26:42

He went away a second time and prayed, "My Father, if it is not possible for this cup to be taken away unless I drink it, may your will be done." NIV

Again he left them and prayed, "My Father! If this cup cannot go away until I drink it all, your will be done." TLB

40 Prayers For Dementia Caregivers

#20 Prayer for Refuge

Oh Lord, how I live for those moments when his eyes twinkle with warmth and remembrance, the smile that plays about his lips. And then, he is gone and I'm left here wondering. Where is he? What is he thinking? What does he see? Heavenly Father, I pray that You keep a tight grasp on his hand. Don't let go. Let him feel Your love and mercy surrounding him. Please, Lord, do not let him feel fearful. Allow him once again to find refuge in Your arms, and I know that I too, will be alright.

Lamentations 3:25-26

The LORD is good to those whose hope is in him,
to the one who seeks him; it is good to wait quietly
for the salvation of the LORD. NIV

The Lord is wonderfully good to those who wait for him, to those who seek for him.
It is good both to hope and wait quietly for the salvation of the Lord. TLB

40 Prayers For Dementia Caregivers

#21 My Fortress

Father, although I complain and perhaps harass you with my unseemly lack of confidence in Your Infinite grace and compassion, I am increasingly aware that this challenge is drawing me near to You. For that I thank you. I am grateful to know that you are beside me.

When I'm discouraged I feel the presence of Your Spirit and I try, Lord, to capture the joy I once knew when my loved one and I could worship You side by side. As I take his hand in mine, I seek your strength for the path ahead, and give you all praise and glory for keeping us close, even at this time of vulnerability.

Psalm 59:16-17

But I will sing of your strength, in the morning I will sing of your love; for you are my fortress, my refuge in times of trouble. You are my strength, I sing praise to you; you, God, are my fortress, my God on whom I can rely. .NIV

But as for me, I will sing each morning about your power and mercy. For you have been my high tower of refuge, a place of safety in the day of my distress. O my Strength, to you I sing my praises; for you are my high tower of safety, my God of mercy. TLB

40 Prayers For Dementia Caregivers

#22 Broaden the Path

We hiked the Grand Canyon together. This path is both narrow and steep. It can also be rocky, dusty, crowded, tedious and long. I wish my feet were like the feet of a deer, able to hoof along sure-footed into high places. If you twist your ankle or get a blister, it will be a long hike out of this canyon. Better to be well prepared. The south rim is 9 miles down- 9 miles up.

There were hours of striving but none to compare with the majesty of reaching the top. Now I have trouble getting you to cross the street carefully. You might hesitate in the middle of the intersection or decide to go back to the side from where you started. I walk in places most people fear to tread in the journey of caring for a loved one with dementia. I never considered preparing for this lifestyle, it has taken me by complete surprise. In the 18th chapter of Psalms, the words say with you Lord, I can scale a wall.

You broaden my path and my ankles do not turn. You can turn darkness into light. I love to hear of your promises. You are the God who arms me with strength.

Psalm 18:33-36

He makes my feet like the feet of a deer; he causes me to stand on the heights. He trains my hands for battle, my arms can bend a bow of bronze. You make your saving help my shield, and your right hand sustains me; your help has made me great. You provide a broad path for my feet, so that my ankles do not give way. NIV

He makes my feet like the feet of a deer; he causes me to stand on the heights. He trains my hands for battle,
my arms can bend a bow of bronze. You make your saving help my shield, and your right hand sustains you're your help has made me great. You provide a broad path for my feet, so that my ankles do not give way. TLB

40 Prayers For Dementia Caregivers

#23 To Feel Whole

I am thankful for all things. If I would not have had the opportunity to be a caregiver, I would not have experienced the ability to feel whole. If life was simple and easy, organized and sweet, would I have called God's name in desperation? Would I have found comfort in my sufficiency rather than cry out to God? Would I ever have learned only God can be my comfort?

Today I thank you for the disease of dementia. Lord it is not always a pretty disease, but I know you dying on the cross was not a pretty happening either. You gave your life away so I could have life in you. Thank you Lord for this mistake that happened in a brain that was at one time healthy. This mistake made me realize my mistake of thinking I was self-sufficient. It is better to be whole with you than half a person with my pride.

Isaiah 66:13

As a mother comforts her child, so will I comfort you NIV

I will comfort you there as a little one is comforted by its mother. TLB

#24 Wasteful Worry

I cannot wear myself out worrying about the day. More harm than good comes from this pattern of thinking. Knowing God calls himself the alpha and omega gives me peace. God wants me to have an abundant life but I never anticipated this lifestyle of dementia caregiving. It can be tedious, discouraging and exhausting. Yet I trust God. He never changes with the happenings of the day or the trends of our culture.

After all He is the creator of the world. From Genesis to Revelations, the bible is full of promises God bestows on those of us who believe in him. He is the beginning and the end, and I will begin this day with his words in my mouth, and end with his word held close to my heart. He is the beginning and the end for all eternity and in my short life. I will strive to speak and think in line with God's word.

Revelations 1:8

I am the Alpha and the Omega, says the Lord God, who is, and who was, and who is to come, the Almighty. NIV

I am the A and the Z, the Beginning and the Ending of all things," says God, who is the Lord, the All Powerful One who is, and was, and is coming again! TLB

Joshua 1:8

Keep this Book of the Law always on your lips; meditate on it day and night, so that you may be careful to do everything written in it. Then you will be prosperous and successful. NIV

Constantly remind the people about these laws, and you yourself must think about them every day and every night so that you will be sure to obey all of them. For only then will you succeed. *TLB*

40 Prayers For Dementia Caregivers

#25 Knit Me Together

We live in a fallen world that is oftentimes unraveling at the edges. But God said he knit me in my mother's womb. God is an orderly God. If you look at nature his ways are precise and orderly. Look at a pinecone, a snowflake, a rose or a majestic oak tree.

If God knit me in my mother's womb would he choose to let me unravel at the seams? If I stay in communication with him, thank him for the things he has given me, and ask for his strength to get through this day, I, too, can thrive in the conditions I live amidst. Lord do not let discouragement creep into my soul. Help me to inspire others to meet challenges with a strength that can only come from you.

Psalm 139:13-14

For you created my inmost being; you knit me together in my mother's womb. I praise you because I am fearfully and wonderfully made; your works are wonderful, I know that full well. NIV

You made all the delicate, inner parts of my body and knit them together in my mother's womb. [14] Thank you for making me so wonderfully complex! It is amazing to think about. Your workmanship is marvelous—and how well I know it. TLB

#26 The Word Holy

The word holy causes me to pause. When the angels sing about God they sang…"Holy, holy, holy." In the days of the scribes, centuries ago, they did not have exclamation points. To make emphasis, they would say or write the word three times. Holy, holy, holy. What a beautiful thought!

Lord help me to develop holiness as I become steadfast in coming to you in prayer. We live in a world of sight and sound, yet you are the small quiet voice, a whisper from within. I need to come to you every day in prayer as it is the best investment of my time. Though I spend such weary hours doing the same thing over and over again for my loved one with dementia, I know you are my best companion. You are wise. You are generous. You are gracious. Above all, you are holy. Holy, holy, holy.

Hebrews 12:10

Our fathers disciplined us for a little while as they thought best; but God disciplines us for our good, that we may share in his holiness. No discipline seems pleasant at the time, but painful. Later on, however, it produces a harvest of righteousness and peace, for those who have been trained by it. NIV

Our earthly fathers trained us for a few brief years, doing the best for us that they knew how, but God's correction is always right and for our best good, that we may share his holiness. TLB

40 Prayers For Dementia Caregivers

#27 My Quiet Time

The television, the computer games, the cell phones, the radio, the newspaper politics, my hobbies - all want to snatch my time away. I need God and my quiet time to be routine. I falter and backslide when I believe I am self-sufficient. With the busyness of caring for one that is dependent on me many hours of the day, I can only find quiet time in small patches.

Still these moments carry me through because if I do not worry and fret, I do not waste my limited energy. I can set all my heavy burdens at your feet. If I am carrying a rock around all day, of course it will get tedious. This is what worry does to me. You have said in your Word, when I am weak, then you are strong. I am relieved to have found my savior who helps me carry my burdens. What a relief! Now… I do not have to do this care giving alone!

2 Corinthians 12:9-10

But he said to me, "My grace is sufficient for you, for my power is made perfect in weakness." Therefore I will boast all the more gladly about my weaknesses, so that Christ's power may rest on me. [10] That is why, for Christ's sake, I delight in weaknesses, in insults, in hardships, in persecutions, in difficulties. For when I am weak, then I am strong. NIV

Each time he said, "No. But I am with you; that is all you need. My power shows up best in weak people." Now I am glad to boast about how weak I am; I am glad to be a living demonstration of Christ's power, instead of showing off my own power and abilities. [10] Since I know it is all for Christ's good, I am quite happy about "the thorn," and about insults and hardships, persecutions and difficulties; for when I am weak, then I am strong—the less I have, the more I depend on him. TLB

40 Prayers For Dementia Caregivers

#28 Less of me, More of You

I love the look of a lighthouse, a beautiful example of a beacon of hope amidst a storm. But if the lighthouse is not built on rock, it would not last long. What if it was built on sand? Without Jesus Christ in our life, it would be like the lighthouse is built on sifting sand. I need a firm foundation or I cannot be strong enough to help my loved one. He has many needs and I cannot be a needy weakling. God has called himself the cornerstone of a building. At times I feel as if my days are unending. What is the outcome of this long term illness? I must be the strong one now. I need an ally.

When I feel fearful, I will look to Jesus as he is my lighthouse. He is the light of the world and his light is my hope. Without hope I am a ship without a rudder, meandering around with no purpose. My day to day happenings generally includes chaos and frustrations but I realize, my help is in the Lord. When I look forward it is not dark, my path is set towards a safe haven in the light. Knowing I am going the right direction makes the journey more enjoyable.

Ephesians 2:19-20

Consequently, you are no longer foreigners and strangers, but fellow citizens with God's people and also members of his household, [20] built on the foundation of the apostles and prophets, with Christ Jesus himself as the chief cornerstone. NIV

Now you are no longer strangers to God and foreigners to heaven, but you are members of God's very own family, citizens of God's country, and you belong in God's household with every other Christian. What a foundation you stand on now: the apostles and the prophets; and the cornerstone of the building is Jesus Christ himself! TLB

40 Prayers For Dementia Caregivers

#29 Yoked to You

Feelings of self pity cause me to feel as if I have a heart of stone instead of a heart of flesh. We safeguard many things but the bible says, above all, safeguard your heart. We change the oil in our cars, we moisturize our face to prevent wrinkles, we keep our portfolio diversified, but what do we do to protect our soul?

Self pity is using energy that is not used in reality but put in a place that is useless. Self pity can cause an insidious leak in the jar that contains all of our good intentions. Lord I give you my feelings of sorrow and focusing on what is not good in my life. I prefer to be yoked to you as you are a strong leader and guide. You know the ways of the world, inside and out, as you designed it, created it and orchestrate it.

How could I ask for a better partner? You know me inside and out. In fact you know me better than I know myself. One of your names is "Ancient of Days." You knew my family from generation to generation. I can breathe a sigh of relief now knowing I have been set free from negative thought patterns. I have asked for forgiveness regarding this and you readily agreed to forgive me. I feel as light as a feather. With this extra energy I am able to be a better care giver for my loved one. I need all the energy I can get as this is considered a long term illness.

Matthew 11:28-29

Come to me, all you who are weary and burdened, and I will give you rest. Take my yoke upon you and learn from me, for I am gentle and humble in heart, and you will find rest for your souls. NIV

Are you tired? Worn out? Burned out on religion? Come to me. Get away with me and you'll recover your life. I'll show you how to take a real rest. Walk with me and work with me—watch how I do it. Learn the unforced rhythms of grace. I won't lay anything heavy or ill-fitting on you. Keep company with me and you'll learn to live freely and lightly. MSG

40 Prayers For Dementia Caregivers

#30 A Contagious Smile

The days turn into weeks, the weeks turn into months, the months turn into seasons, and before long the year has ended. We can bring our days to God and he will put them in his very capable hands. Then we simply do the next things. It is as simple as that! When I am in communion with God I am amazed at the plan he has for my day. If I am in tune to his ways, I am on the outlook for ways to please him.

One small thing after another and if I do the small things well, the big things take care of themselves. "I am with you. I am with you." God must be chanting this in my ear. I can sense his presence. I chant back…"I trust you. I trust you." I feel a harmony that I have not experienced in weeks, months, seasons, and years. I smile, and when I smile, my loved one generally smiles back. Though the memory is impaired, the ability to smile is a basic component that is, as of yet, not lost. It is a small joy that I relish.

Isaiah 61:7

Instead of your shame you will receive a double portion, and instead of disgrace you will rejoice in your inheritance. And so you will inherit a double portion in your land, and everlasting joy will be yours. NIV

Messages of joy instead of news of doom, a praising heart instead of a languid spirit. Rename them "Oaks of Righteousness" planted by GOD to display his glory. They'll rebuild the old ruins, raise a new city out of the wreckage. They'll start over on the ruined cities, take the rubble left behind and make it new. You'll hire outsiders to herd your flocks and foreigners to work your fields, But you'll have the title "Priests of GOD," honored as ministers of our God. You'll feast on the bounty of nations, you'll bask in their glory. Because you got a double dose of trouble and more than your share of contempt, Your inheritance in the land will be doubled and your joy go on forever. TLB

#31 Obedience to God

Noah demonstrated leadership strength in his obedience to God. A verse in the Bible "Noah did everything just as God had commanded him" is easy to read and skip over. But every word is important in the Bible. Noah did 'everything' as God commanded him – not some things. I read the Bible and believe what is written, but, Lord, it is another thing to act upon what I read. Noah listened to what You said and then actually did it. Noah's obedience is a lesson for all leaders because of the massive task given to him. With little help Noah spent 120 years building an enormous ark in an area where water never came from the heavens (rain). I am grateful, Lord, that You teach me through stories about leaders in the Bible. Let me listen and obey your call for wherever and whatever situation you want to bring me into this life. I want to be like Noah – to hear and obey.

Genesis 6:22 to 7:1

Noah did everything just as God commanded him. The Lord then said to Noah, "Go into the ark, you and your whole family, because I have found you righteous in this generation." NIV

And Noah did everything as God commanded him. Finally the day came when the Lord said to Noah, "Go into the boat with all your family, for among all the people of the earth, I consider you alone to be righteous. TLB

40 Prayers For Dementia Caregivers

#32 Call to Me

God, help me to call to You during these tough times. When doubt tempts me to believe that what is happening is unfair and my self-pity and anxiety swells, remind me that those unsearchable things that I do not know will be revealed to me all in Your timing. Help me Lord to call to You for help. Especially when caring for my loved one, I do not want to question your providence. I will trust your plan!

Jeremiah 33:2-3

"This is what the LORD says, he who made the earth, the LORD who formed it and established it—the LORD is his name: 'Call to me and I will answer you and tell you great and unsearchable things you do not know.' NIV

The Lord, the Maker of heaven and earth—Jehovah is his name—says this: Ask me and I will tell you some remarkable secrets about what is going to happen here.
TLB

#33 When I am Weak, I am Strong

Lord Jesus, I am not sure why you have me going down this path. All around me it seems I'm being tested. The difficulties often feel too challenging. Please help strengthen me to serve. Please strengthen me to follow Your direction and leadership. Please Lord open my eyes to Your power and let the weaknesses that I have completely fade away. Help me to persevere to pray daily.

Matthew 26:41

"Watch and pray so that you will not fall into temptation. The spirit is willing, but the flesh is weak." "Watch and pray so that you will not fall into temptation. The spirit is willing, but the flesh is weak." NIV

Keep alert and pray. Otherwise temptation will overpower you. For the spirit indeed is willing, but how weak the body is!" TLB

40 Prayers For Dementia Caregivers

#34 Wait!

Lord, I want to take responsibility for the things I see that need to change. I know you are greater than all of these things. I know You understand the reason this is happening. Please help me to wait on You and be renewed. When I am weary I visualize flying in the blue sky on an Eagles wing! You are that eagle, Lord Jesus.

Isaiah 40:31

But those who hope in the LORD
will renew their strength.
They will soar on wings like eagles;
they will run and not grow weary,
they will walk and not be faint. NIV

But they that wait upon the Lord shall renew their strength. They shall mount up with wings like eagles; they shall run and not be weary; they shall walk and not faint. TLB

40 Prayers For Dementia Caregivers

#35 God is For Us!

Lord Jesus. You died on the cross for my sins. Thank You!
There is nothing on earth than I desire more than You.
At times I feel as if there are so many things against me -
the difficult time caring for my loved one, the extended family and all their concerns,
the medical staff, and most of the time my own negative self talk.

Please help me to remember that God is for me,
He is in control. No matter what difficulty I encounter,
If God is for me, who can be against me?

Romans 8:31-37

What, then, shall we say in response to these things? If God is for us, who can be against us? He who did not spare his own Son, but gave him up for us all—how will he not also, along with him, graciously give us all things? Who will bring any charge against those whom God has chosen? It is God who justifies. Who then is the one who condemns? No one. Christ Jesus who died—more than that, who was raised to life—is at the right hand of God and is also interceding for us. Who shall separate us from the love of Christ? Shall trouble or hardship or persecution or famine or nakedness or danger or sword? As it is written:

*"For your sake we face death all day long;
we are considered as sheep to be slaughtered."*

No, in all these things we are more than conquerors through him who loved us. NIV

What can we ever say to such wonderful things as these? If God is on our side, who can ever be against us? Since he did not spare even his own Son for us but gave him up for us all, won't he also surely give us everything else? Who dares accuse us whom God has chosen for his own? Will God? No! He is the one who has forgiven us and given us right standing with himself. Who then will condemn us? Will Christ? No! For he is the one who died for us and came back to life again for us *and is sitting at the place of highest honor next to God, pleading for us there in heaven. Who then can ever keep Christ's love from us? When we have trouble or calamity, when we are hunted down or destroyed, is it because he doesn't love us anymore? And if we are hungry or penniless or in danger or threatened with death, has God deserted us? No, for the Scriptures tell us that for his sake we must be ready to face death at every moment of the day—we are like sheep awaiting slaughter; ³⁷ but despite all this, overwhelming victory is ours through Christ who loved us enough to die for us. TLB*

40 Prayers For Dementia Caregivers

#36 Where Does My Help Come From

Jesus, I sometimes question Your promises and Your plan. Please help me to realize that everything comes from You! I know that my help and strength come from You, Lord Jesus! You watch over me and provide solid ground upon which I walk. Help me follow You wherever You lead. Although I feel so helpless in the situations that I am facing. I know You are standing with me. My heart is tempted to get hardened towards You, yet I know this a place for where I can witness about your goodness. Please guide me. Your unending love and grace inspires me to develop endurance.

Psalm 121:1-8

I lift up my eyes to the mountains—
where does my help come from?
My help comes from the LORD,
the Maker of heaven and earth.

He will not let your foot slip—
he who watches over you will not slumber;
indeed, he who watches over Israel
will neither slumber nor sleep.

The LORD watches over you—
the LORD is your shade at your right hand;
the sun will not harm you by day,
nor the moon by night.

The LORD will keep you from all harm—
he will watch over your life;
the LORD will watch over your coming and going
both now and forevermore. NIV

Shall I look to the mountain gods for help? No! My help is from Jehovah who made the mountains! And the heavens too! He will never let me stumble, slip, or fall. For he is always watching, never sleeping. Jehovah himself is caring for you! He is your defender. He protects you day and night. He keeps you from all evil and preserves your life. He keeps his eye upon you as you come and go and always guards you. TLB

40 Prayers For Dementia Caregivers

#37 God Provides

Lord! Jesus! God, You are the creator of all things. You provide for us in all situations. From our vantage point, we may not have complete understanding of why You allow these things to happen, but we accept Your will is supreme. You will continue to provide for us in Your timing. You are the sustainer of all life. You make it so I am satisfied. Thank You, Lord. My cup overflows.

2 Kings 4:1-7

The wife of a man from the company of the prophets cried out to Elisha, "Your servant my husband is dead, and you know that he revered the LORD. But now his creditor is coming to take my two boys as his slaves." Elisha replied to her, "How can I help you? Tell me, what do you have in your house?" "Your servant has nothing there at all," she said, "except a small jar of olive oil." Elisha said, "Go around and ask all your neighbors for empty jars. Don't ask for just a few. Then go inside and shut the door behind you and your sons. Pour oil into all the jars, and as each is filled, put it to one side." She left him and shut the door behind her and her sons. They brought the jars to her and she kept pouring. When all the jars were full, she said to her son, "Bring me another one." But he replied, "There is not a jar left." Then the oil stopped flowing. She went and told the man of God, and he said, "Go, sell the oil and pay your debts. You and your sons can live on what is left."
NIV

One day the wife of one of the seminary students came to Elisha to tell him of her husband's death. He was a man who had loved God, she said. But he had owed some money when he died, and now the creditor was demanding it back. If she didn't pay, he said he would take her two sons as his slaves. "What shall I do?" Elisha asked. "How much food do you have in the house?" "Nothing at all, except a jar of olive oil," she replied. "Then borrow many pots and pans from your friends and neighbors!" he instructed. ⁴ "Go into your house with your sons and shut the door behind you. Then pour olive oil from your jar into the pots and pans, setting them aside as they are filled!" So she did. Her sons brought the pots and pans to her, and she filled one after another! ⁶ Soon every container was full to the brim" "Bring me another jar," she said to her sons. "There aren't any more!" they told her. And then the oil stopped flowing! When she told the prophet what had happened, he said to her, "Go and sell the oil and pay your debt, and there will be enough money left for you and your sons to live on!" TLB

#38 The Lord, the Great Physician

Jesus, please let me do what is right. Lord Jesus, I pray that my eyes be continually focused on You. I pray that You would guide my care-giving decisions so they please You. Please help me to put You first in all things. May I use my healing hands for Your glory. Other people come to me with their stressful and sorrowful stories. I want to help, but Lord, I have sorrows and sins of my own. But with You I am able to listen and be compassionate.

Please help me to be content with the fruit I bear and the harvest You provide.

I praise You Lord with all I have. You are my great Physician.

Matthew 9:12

"On hearing this, Jesus said, "It is not the healthy who need a doctor, but the sick." NIV

Because people who are well don't need a doctor! It's the sick people who do!" was Jesus' reply. TLB

40 Prayers For Dementia Caregivers

#39 A Cheerful Heart

Lord, please help me to have a cheerful heart in all circumstances, especially when I have to perform difficult tasks for my loved one about their personal needs. Help me to be a light to him or her as You would be. Help me to provide my loved one with the good medicine of a cheerful heart. When I fix my eyes on You, I am joyful.

Proverbs 17:22

A cheerful heart is good medicine, but a crushed spirit dries up the bones. NIV

A cheerful heart does good like medicine, but a broken spirit makes one sick. TLB

40 Prayers For Dementia Caregivers

#40 Guide Me, O Lord

Lord, help me to work more on my soul than my health. Please allow me to be able to serve with love and compassion. Help me to hold steadfast to the goals You have set out for us in Your word. Lord, please help me to encourage others in whatever physical or spiritual turmoil they may be battling. Please Lord Jesus, I love You and cherish You above all things.

3 John 2

Dear friend, I pray that you may enjoy good health and that all may go well with you, even as your soul is getting along well. NIV

Dear friend, I am praying that all is well with you and that your body is as healthy as I know your soul is. TLB

About The Authors

Diane McGiffin is a wife, mother of one grown daughter, sister, friend, recently retired licensed nurse and art museum docent. This past year Diane moved from Scottsdale, Arizona to Kalamazoo, Michigan to be closer to her family.

For over ten years she was a charge nurse of a dementia unit in Scottsdale and has developed firsthand insight when helping those with dementia and the family, loved ones and staff, that cared for them. Many of the stories shared are from her memory of caregivers expressing these very thoughts and concerns as she worked in the dementia unit as a nurse.

Marlene Graeve is a registered nurse with a Bachelor's Degree in business management. She has worked in pediatrics, assisted living and long term care, home health care, dementia units, and hospice inpatient care. She has earned certifications in gerontological nursing, hospice, and palliative care. She is presently employed at Superior Home Health Care in Lakeville, Minnesota.

Marlene is married, has 3 grown children, and 7 grandchildren. Marlene lives in Minneapolis and loves to vacation in Scottsdale, Arizona. She published the article "The Dementia Dozen: 12 tips for Alzheimer's Disease Caregivers" in Minnesota Health Care News Magazine.

D. Duane Engler is a son, husband, father of three boys. He coaches his son's hockey and soccer. He loves the Lord and strives to work for Jesus in all he does.

As a professional educator and speaker D. Duane aims to help others live out Proverbs 4:26 as they consider the paths of their feet. He lives in Edina, Minnesota, where he is working on his next book.

Scripture Meditation and Prayer

You will see Me and you will find Me when you search for Me with all your heart.
Jeremiah 29:13 NIV

FIND a private location and open your Bible to the Scripture for meditation and prayer. Use the same location every day, if possible, and at the same time so it will become a daily habit. You might consider mornings when your mind is fresh. If just starting out, meditate and pray for 15 minutes. You will find yourself wanting more time as you develop a closer relationship with God. Kneel down as you pray if physically able.

But when you pray, go into your room, close the door and pray to your Father, who is unseen. Then your Father, who sees what is done in secret, will reward you.
Matthew 6:6 NIV

CLOSE your eyes – calm your mind. Focus on your breath or Bible verse (examples: Psalm 46:10 or use a verse to memorize) to clear your mind from worldly thoughts.

"Be still and know that I am God..." Psalm 46:10 NIV

ASK God for His favor as you meditate and pray.

May these words of my mouth and this meditation of my heart be pleasing in your sight, Lord, my Rock and my Redeemer. Psalm 19:14 NIV

ALLOW the Holy Spirit to speak to you through the Scripture.

But the Advocate, the Holy Spirit whom the Father will send in my name, will teach you all things and will remind you of everything I have said to you. John 14:26 NIV

WORSHIP - Holy, Holy, Holy, Lord, God Almighty

Lord, our Lord, how majestic is your name in all the earth! Psalm 8:9 NIV

How great you are, Sovereign Lord! There is no one like You, and there is no God but You, as we have heard with our own ears. 2 Samuel 7:22 NIV

CONFESS your sins to cleanse your heart.

Then I acknowledged my sin to you and did not cover up my iniquity. I said, "I will confess my transgressions to the Lord." And you forgave the guilt of my sin. Psalm 32:5 NIV

PRAY the Lord's Prayer and your personal devotions, requests, thanksgiving, intercessory prayers, etc.

This, then, is how you should pray: "Our Father in heaven, hallowed by your name, your kingdom come, your will be done, or earth as it is in heaven. Give us today our daily bread. And forgive us our debts, as we also have forgiven our debtors. And lead us not into temptation, but deliver us from the evil one. Matthew 6:9-13 NIV

Meditation Recommendations:

READ the chosen Scripture several times. Each time reflect on the meaning of the Scripture, relating it specifically to you and your relationship with Jesus.

1. Change the words in the Bible verse around as if you are talking to God in the first person (use the words I, me, we, and our). Commit to memorize one or two Bible verses a month.

2. Slowly read the verse several times -- each time emphasize a different word: **I** meditate on Your precepts; I **meditate** on Your precepts; I meditate on **Your** precepts, I meditate on Your **precepts**…

3. Ask the Holy Spirit, "What does this verse mean for me?" Be quiet and wait for an answer, thought, or direction to another Bible verse.

4. If you are discouraged or feel helpless and confused by the Scripture and the Holy Spirit is quiet – stay calm and ask God to bring something or someone into your life that week that will help you understand the Scripture more clearly.

I meditate on Your precepts and consider Your ways. Psalm 119:15 NIV

THANK God with heartfelt thanksgiving.

Give thanks to the Lord, for He is good; His love endures forever. 1 Chronicles 16:34 NIV

All this is for your benefit, so that the grace that is reaching more and more people may cause thanksgiving to overflow to the glory of God. 2 Corinthians 4:15 NIV

Author's Section on Prayer and the 40 Prayers™ Series:

What is Christian prayer?

Prayer is communication with God. Communicating with Him from our place of weakness, surrender, and vulnerability so He would work in our lives, strengthening us for the tasks He has called us to do. Prayer is asking Him for guidance and skills that would allow us to honor Him more. Prayer is thanksgiving,

Prayer has been defined as an utterance, fervent request, entreaty, devout petition, praise, thanks, beseech, or crave. While the Internet provides many definitions of prayer, let's review vital points about prayer from a Christian perspective.

Is Christian prayer cross-cultural?

Christian prayer is cross-cultural and universal. God put the need for prayer in everyone's heart. Open Christian prayer is easier is some countries than others. Prayer to Jesus Chris is: (1) open and non-restricted, (2) monitored, (3) hostile, or (4) restricted depending on the country you live in or visit.

A Christian organization (The Voice of the Martyrs at www.persecution.com) defines these categories:

"Monitored areas are being closely monitored by some Christian organizations because of a trend toward increased Christian persecution. Hostile includes nations or large areas of nations where governments consistently attempt to provide protection for the Christian populations but where Christians are routinely persecuted by family friends, neighbors or political groups because of their witness. Restricted includes countries where government-sanctioned circumstances or anti-Christian laws lead to Christians being harassed, imprisoned, killed, or deprived of possessions or liberties because of their witnesses. This includes countries where government policy or practice prevents Christians from obtaining Bibles or other Christian literature."

The "God need" that is in our heart can only be filled by Him. Regardless of where you are or what country you are in, God knows your prayers even when prayer is not spoken out loud.

Who should pray?

Everyone. Christ calls us to pray to Him in all things for He is the way, the truth, and the life. No one comes to the Father except through Him. Start as early as possible praying with young children. The evil one knows he can tempt young children so you must start prayer early. You can even pray for children you want to have or the child that is in the womb.

Does God answer every prayer?

Pray and meditate on these verses regarding answered prayer:

1 John 5:14-15 *"That is the confidence we have in approaching God: that if we ask anything according to his will, He hears us. And if we know that He hears us – whatever we ask – we know that we have what we asked of him."* NIV

John 15:16 *"You did not choose me, but I chose you and appointed you so that you might go and bear fruit – fruit that will last – and so that whatever you ask in my name the Father will give you."* NIV

Matthew 7:7 *"Ask and it will be given to you; seek and you will find; knock and the door will be opened to you."* NIV

Romans 8:28 *"And we know that in all things God works for the good of those who love him, who have been called according to his purpose."* NIV

Isaiah 59:2 *"But your iniquities have separated you from your God; your sins have hidden His face from you, so that He will not hear."* NIV

If we go to God, but we are not in a right place with Him, what shall we do?

Ask God to prepare your heart to receive His Word. Read your Bible. Confess your sins. Ask a pastor or friend to seek direction by praying with them to God.

Where and when can we pray?

Anywhere and anytime. You do not need to close your eyes or be on your knees. On the other hand, you can close your eyes throughout your prayer and spend the entire time on your knees. Prayer happens in your heart and your mind. Keep in constant communication with him formally each morning or night and informally throughout the day. He is always there waiting for you.

What should we pray about?

Anything. Talk to Jesus as you would a friend. Tell Him what is on your mind, what you are concerned about, what you need help with. Thank Him and honor Him every time you pray. Ask Him for guidance and direction. Pray for your family and loved ones. Pray for people you do not even know by name. Your prayers can be big or small.

If God has full control and knows how things will end up, why then do we still pray?

We pray because He told us to do it. In Matthew 7:7, we are told to ask, seek, and knock. It's that simple.

Matthew 7:7 *"Ask and it will be given to you; seek and you will find; knock and the door will be opened to you."* NIV

How should we pray?

Many people who pray use the acronym "ACTS". ACTS stands for Adoration, Confession, Thanksgiving, and Supplication (which is a way of asking God for something). Do not worry if you are not sure which category your prayer fits in to or the full meaning of supplication. The reality is that God honors any sincere prayer.

As I am not an English major please forgive any grammatical or syntax errors in the prayers. When you pray, God does not care about the grammar or structure of your prayer. He just wants your heart; please give it to Him.

What type of application can you take from the 40 Prayers™ Series?

Application questions surrounding prayers and Bible verses are the most fun as it convicts my soul. Conviction draws me closer to the peace of walking with Jesus Christ. Consider these questions when you pray and read Bible verses:

1. What did this Scripture mean when it was written?
An application Bible may be helpful – you can buy online or in any Christian bookstore.

2. What does this Scripture mean for me today?
Reflect on what comes to your mind or what you are convicted by the Holy Spirit.

3. How can I apply this Scripture to my life?
What specifically is happening in your life where this Scripture fits?

4. What should I start doing, stop doing, or change?
Is there anyone who God has put on my heart that I should share this with?

If you need additional prayer, help, or assistance where can you go or whom can you contact?

Your local church or a trusted specific ministry is a good place to start for support. The issues you face will significantly benefit from prayer. Greater professional, medical, or pastoral support may be needed. Honor and respect your body, and do not be afraid to ask for help,

Why the 40 Prayers™ Series?

The 40 Prayers™ Series is a simple focus of prayer and action. The format is a topic, heartfelt prayer, and supporting verse. The intention is for the books to be easy to access and read with devotional prayer for anyone, anywhere, and anytime. The prayers are filled with meaningful application with a biblical grounding and focus on Christ.

What is the focus of the 40 Prayers™ Series Ministry?

1. Spark a revival in the lives of people through prayer to Jesus Christ
2. Reach others with the message of Christ's redeeming sacrifice of dying on the cross for our sins
3. Explain how to be productive, intentional, and resourceful with the gifts God has given us
4. Understand the need for prayer in our world

40 Prayers™ Series was started after numerous prayers on direction and application of God's truth in our life and the reality of God's sovereignty. Forty (40) is a significant number in the Bible that means complete or completion. With these prayers my hope is that you would begin, develop, or enhance your relationship with Jesus Christ.

With the desire to leave a legacy of prayer for my family and children, I decided to retain my prayers for them in a written format. When a friend suggested I memorialize these prayers, I decided to publish them. After my death, my children will realize how important prayer was in their father's life. Hopefully, more than my immediate family will benefit from this series. My prayer is that these books would inspire you to pray, to grasp God's unconditional love and underserving grace, to bring people to accept Jesus Christ as their Savior, and to encourage and comfort others in need.

Many times in speaking with people we say we will pray for them or we write this in a greeting card. We end up neglecting that prayer time because we forget or are too busy. The 40 Prayers™ Series is something tangible you can send a friend or family member during life's needs, challenges, and celebrations, always keeping the focus on prayer.

I see a need for spiritual revival in our hearts, families, communities, and our world. Revival starts with prayer. As God as our sovereign Lord, if enough people reach out to Him in prayer, who knows what the outcomes could be. But He knows!

What can you do to support the 40 Prayers™ Series?

If you feel compelled, write a review where you purchased the book or recommend the 40 Prayer Series to others. That would be very gracious. You can bless one of your friends or family members with a copy. The book may bring him or her one step closer to accepting Christ as Savior.

We appreciate your support and fellowship through this prayer ministry. If you are feeling led to translate a book into another language, please let me know as we are in need of translators to reach others around the world. If you have ideas to benefit others through the 40 Prayers Series ministry or to reach more people, please let us know.

Let's rock the world with prayer!

May you live your life as a prayer honoring Christ Jesus in everything. To our precious Lord Jesus Christ is the glory!

Many blessings,

D. Duane Engler

James 1:2-12

"Consider it pure joy, my brothers and sisters, whenever you face trials of many kinds, ³ because you know that the testing of your faith produces perseverance. Let perseverance finish its work so that you may be mature and complete, not lacking anything. If any of you lacks wisdom, you should ask God, who gives generously to all without finding fault, and it will be given to you. But when you ask, you must believe and not doubt, because the one who doubts is like a wave of the sea, blown and tossed by the wind. That person should not expect to receive anything from the Lord. Such a person is double-minded and unstable in all they do.

Believers in humble circumstances ought to take pride in their high position. But the rich should take pride in their humiliation—since they will pass away like a wild flower. For the sun rises with scorching heat and withers the plant; its blossom falls and its beauty is destroyed. In the same way, the rich will fade away even while they go about their business.

Blessed is the one who perseveres under trial because, having stood the test, that person will receive the crown of life that the Lord has promised to those who love him." NIV